When You're
The Caregiver

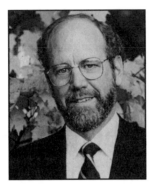

Jim Miller combines several professions and various interests in his work at Willowgreen. He is an ordained clergyman, having served in the pastoral ministry for sixteen years, and a grief counselor. As a writer, photographer, and video producer he has produced a number of books and videotapes in the areas of loss and grief, transition, older age, caregiving, and spirituality. Jim also creates his own multi-media presentations for use in his workshops, seminars, and speeches. He regularly presents his award-winning work before many regional and national groups.

To learn about his speaking schedule or to inquire about his availability to present before your group, contact

Willowgreen Publishing
10351 Dawson's Creek Boulevard, Suite B
Fort Wayne, Indiana 46825
260-490-2222

When You're The Caregiver

12 Things To Do If Someone You Care for Is Ill or Incapacitated

James E. Miller

Willowgreen Publishing

This book grows out of the generosity of several wonderful people who shared their ideas and their feedback unselfishly. They include John VanderZee, Micheline Sommers, John Peterson, Bernie Miller, Jennifer Levine, Jim Kragness, Gail Kittleson, Carrie Hackney, Dick Gilbert, John Gantt, Patricia Ferro, Bob Dexter, Jeana Bodart, Clare Barton, and John Aleshire.

❀

Willowgreen Publishing
10351 Dawson's Creek Boulevard, Suite B
Fort Wayne, Indiana 46825
260-490-2222

Library of Congress Catalogue
Card Number: 95-90163

ISBN 1-885933-21-5

You may have become a caregiver only recently, or you may have begun a long time ago. You may have taken on this role temporarily, or you may expect to have it as long as both you and the one for whom you are caring are alive. The two of you may live under the same roof, or you may not. You may be close, or you may be at a distance. This experience may be a labor of love, or a labor of loss, or a labor of obligation, or hardly a labor at all.

Whatever your situation, you know that being a caregiver can be a demanding task. Our society idealizes self-sufficiency, yet the very nature of your circumstances may require you to turn to others for help. Your caregiving responsibilities may consume you, absorbing your time and your psychological energy and your physical stamina. You may find yourself overstretched, trying to handle commitments to your job, or to other family members, or to yourself, or, as is often the case, to all the above. You may feel ill-prepared to assume your role, or ill-equipped, or ill-suited.

It's quite possible you may have a different response: you may feel gratified you can help and quite confident of your abilities. Your concerns may be few.

This book is written for all of you. Because no two situations and no two caregiving relationships are exactly alike, the twelve suggestions presented here are general in nature. Adapt them to fit your individual circumstances. Pass over some ideas and expand others. Do what's right for you. You'll know.

❀

1
Be with your feelings.

You may be inclined to focus on the needs and the feelings of the one you're caring for, at the expense of your own. That can be a natural reaction, especially as you begin this relationship, and especially if the other person is suffering. You want to do what you can and you would like to make things right for the other. So you may suppress your own emotions in order to carry out your responsibilities.

Be aware: suppressing your emotions in the short run can be an act of love, but suppressing them over the long haul is a serious mistake.

There are no prescribed feelings for you to have. Everyone experiences a time like this a little differently. No two people feel the same emotions, in the same sequence, with the same intensity. So don't program your-self for what you will feel, and don't let others program you either.

Following are some of the reactions that caregivers commonly report early in the process:

• *Shock and confusion,* sometimes including wondering if you're going a little crazy.

• *Anxiety and fear,* about what is happening now or what may happen in the future.

• *Sadness or depression,* especially if the situation seems overwhelming or discouraging.

• *Anger,* perhaps toward these circumstances, or the person you're caring for, or whatever or whoever may have caused these events. You may be mad at yourself, or at people who are less than helpful right now, or at God.

• *Guilt,* about what you have done or not done.

• *Grief,* for what the other person has lost, and perhaps what you have lost as well. These losses may be visible and distinct, or they may be hard to pinpoint but no less real.

The range and depth of your feelings will be related to your relationship with the other person, the seriousness of their condition, the impact this situation will have on your life, and many other factors. This experience may affect you very deeply, more deeply than you might have imagined.

At the same time, you may find you don't have as much support for your own feelings as you would like. People may be so concerned for the one who is ill or incapacitated that they forget you need attention as well.

As your caregiving duties expand, other feelings may develop:

• *Frustration and irritability*, with so many pressures, demands, disappointments.

• *Loneliness*, as family and friends go about their lives without you.

• *Shame*, for the other's condition, or for how you're responding, or for needing help.

• *Helplessness*, for all the things you cannot do for the other.

• *Exhaustion*, on any level: physical, mental, psychological, or spiritual.

Of course, you may have other more cheerful emotions, too:

• *Joy*, in being with the other.

• *Gratitude*, for what you've been given.

• *Pride*, in what you've been able to do.

• *Love*, for all the obvious reasons.

Remember that all of your feelings are valid. Feelings are not right or wrong. They are simply signs that you're human, that you're engaged in life, that you care. So do what all healthy caregivers do: feel fully whatever it is you feel.

❀

2
Express your feelings.

Feeling your emotions is the first step. But it's only a step. You dare not stop there. Your feelings need to be freed somehow. One of your responsibilities as a mature caregiver is to find ways to make that happen.

Only you can determine how much you will express to the person in your care. Probably you will want them to know at least certain things: your concern, your affection, and your confidence in them. If your caregiving relationship began suddenly with a crisis, or if that person is seriously ill, it will be wise to spare them all that is happening to you, at least for the time being. They have plenty to deal with already.

Are there other family members with whom you can share? Are there close friends who will support you? If you're in a hospital setting, what about a chaplain or a social worker or a visiting clergyperson? Sometimes doctors and nurses have pockets of time to spend with you. Sometimes you can find willing ears where you may not expect them: visiting acquaintances, hospital volunteers, even perfect strangers who happen to be perfect listeners.

Face-to-face talking helps, because you can communicate with more than just your words. But you can also connect with others across telephone lines and even through computer terminals, or with handwritten letters or homemade recordings. It's not important <u>how</u> you do it. It's simply important that you <u>do</u> it. Having at least one other human being know what you're going through and what you're feeling can be quite therapeutic.

As time goes by, you may find other outlets for your feelings: perhaps a support group for caregivers like yourself, or a regularly-scheduled luncheon with a few friends, or appointments with a professional counselor. You may find you don't know what you feel until you begin talking. That's another reason why it's so important.

You can express your feelings in other ways, of course. Journaling is a means of letting go of your emotions and saving them at the same time. You may find you'll learn a lot by reading back over what you've written. Some people put their words into songs or poems or prayers–perhaps you're one.

Of course, you may choose not to use words at all. Have you ever tried drawing or painting or photographing your feelings? What about ventilating them with a good yell or a great cry? A friend I know vents her anger by stomping on inverted styrofoam cups or by throwing eggs at trees. Another releases her feelings by sewing. Another plays the violin.

However you express yourself, it's vital that you do so. Any time you are in a close relationship with another, your feelings come into play. Any time you are living through a momentous or stress-filled time, your feelings will be stronger than normal. And any time you do not find ways to express your strong feelings, they will come out in their own unique ways–perhaps ways you would not yourself choose.

❀

3
Listen. Just listen.

The person you're caring for needs to do exactly what you need to do. They usually need to talk about what is going on, and express their feelings, and communicate both their fears and their hopes. In other words, they need to tell their story. As often as not, they need not only to tell it, but to re-tell it. And maybe even re-tell it again.

People who are ill or injured or somehow disabled deserve to have someone witness what is happening to them. It validates their own importance and the importance of this episode in their life. It may help to ease their suffering. It may have a way of putting things in perspective.

The emotions they choose to share with you may be strong ones. These may be painful to express, and just as painful to hear. But this joint act of telling and witnessing can help make these feelings more manageable. It can help make this time more stable, and the other's outlook more positive.

Allow the other person to speak whatever their feelings are. Help them appreciate that feelings are not to be judged one way or another. They are to be accepted as charges of energy that flow through you. Your feelings show how much you care, how much you're involved in life, how much things matter to you.

To be a good listener, try some of these ideas:

• Place yourself on the other's eye level, so you're communicating as equals.

• Be close enough so you can speak comfortably without raising your voice.

• Keep distractions to a minimum: objects that come between you, interruptions by others, sights or sounds that divert your attention.

• Hold the other person in your gaze rather than often looking away.

• Nod and give verbal cues that you have heard.

• Ask questions if you don't grasp something.

• Touch the other, if it seems appropriate and if it is okay with them. Holding the other's hand or touching their wrist or arm or shoulder can comfort them and connect you both.

• Briefly summarize important thoughts and rephrase significant feelings in order to get as close as you can to your understanding of what the other person said, and to let the other know you <u>do</u> understand.

• Remember that silence can be a way of speaking. Allow the other to be quiet when they wish, and allow yourself to be quiet, too.

How you listen may determine how the other will speak. If you're hurried, if you judge what they're saying, if you'd rather not be there, the other person will know it. They may then restrict what they will expose to you.

If you're like many, you may say to yourself, "This isn't much—I'm doing nothing more than listening." Banish those thoughts. Realize that listening is one of the most life-giving and life-affirming gifts you can offer another, especially when the other is ill or hurting. Your accepting, listening presence encourages the other person to become more whole.

❀

4
Communicate with the one you care for.
Really communicate.

By its very nature, hospitalization can be dehumanizing. Consider how hospital gowns look and feel. How rooms are often sterile (in order to be sterilized, if needed). How regulations and paperwork can overshadow the personal dimension. A long convalesence at home or an unending illness anywhere can be disorienting and isolating. An unwanted disability can be infuriating and discombobulating.

You can be a lifeline to sanity in the way you communicate.

• *Offer honest communication.* When one's sense of security has been disrupted, when life seems up for grabs, people need to trust in something or someone. Ideally, one of those "someones" will be you. Ideally, you can assure them with your honesty.

Chances are you won't be saying everything you're thinking and feeling–circumstances don't call for that. But generally, it's best to be truthful in whatever you do say. Deceiving the other about medical reports or prognoses puts a wedge between the two of you and destroys trust. It prevents the other from confirming their own feelings, from being able to re-direct their energies, or from making well-informed decisions about the way they live their days.

Be straightforward about the other's desires and needs. Ask how you can best help, rather than presuming you know. Learn about the specific things they like, and the things they don't. Inquire about the ways your caregiving limits them, and how it frees them, and how it affirms them. Ask them for their honesty as you give them yours.

• *Offer sensitive communication.* By all that you say and all that you don't, let the other know you're open to their feelings as well as their wonderings and their reasonings.

Accept their deepest sentiments. As the time is right, and if the situation calls for it, you may wish to share your own.

There may be occasions for tears. Allow them to come, whether they belong to the other or to you. Sometimes mingled tears create the most endearing bonds of all, as well as the most meaningful lessons.

• *Offer entertaining communication.* At times the one who is ill or incapacitated needs diversions, or light-hearted conversation, or news of the outside world. Look for topics that will lift the other's spirits and expand the other's horizons. Follow their lead.

• *Avoid certain types of communication.* Some things you say may get in the way of bonding with the other. Platitudes can create a distance between you, especially those words that don't ring true. "I know exactly how you feel" may <u>sound</u> comforting, but the truth is you can't and you don't. "This will make you a better person" is empty consolation when one is deep in pain. "God never gives you more than you can handle" is a hollow thought if the other is feeling desperate.

Advice, especially if it's unsolicited, can sound judgmental or parental. Awkward, forced cheerfulness will quickly limit what the other can talk about. Attempts to minimize the other's condition or to downplay the other's feelings can drive them away, and so can excessive talk about your own discomforts or problems.

In general, communicate about anything that is important or interesting or entertaining to both of you. But really communicate.

❀

5
Treat the other as the equal he or she is.

The unfortunate truth is this: the other's injury or illness or disability may become such a focus it almost replaces the rest of their identity. This process, initiated by family and friends as well as by professionals and strangers, is often unintentional and unconscious. But it is not unimportant. It is a destructive act.

The tendency to diminish and dehumanize the other occurs in various ways. You may make decisions for them without bothering to consult them. Or you may treat them as helpless by doing things they are capable of doing on their own, things they even wish to do. You may use infantile language, as in, "What are we going to wear today, dear?" You may find yourself feeling pity rather than empathy.

Never forget: the person you're caring for is just as unique and just as complex as before. They are just as sacred as ever. And that person deserves to be respected and treated as such. Ask yourself: if <u>you</u> do not treat them as a valued equal, who will?

Some ways you can be conscious of relating to the other as an equal include:

• Expect the other to maintain as much control over their life as they wish and as they are able. Support them in this.

• Validate what you esteem in the other by what you say and do. Make sure the other knows what you respect about them.

• If the other has changed a great deal as a result of this experience, look beneath the surface and treasure their heart and soul.

• Be accepting of the other's place on their journey, even if it's not where you believe you would be. For starters, you can't know for sure how you would respond in the same situation. In addition, it's not your role to change the other person. Only they can do that.

Relating to the other as your equal is healthy, but it is not always easy to do. The other may not agree with you–and has that right. The other may get angry–and has that freedom. The other may test you and try to alienate you, to see how committed you are to staying with them. The other may take out their frustrations on you, when they're really upset about something else. You may be a "safe target," or the only target available to them.

When you have times of strain, here are some ways to handle it:

• Honestly look to see if you have been treating the other as less than equal, even in small ways. If you have, admit it. Then strive to change.

• Visualize yourself in the other's situation. Ask yourself what <u>you</u> might feel, how <u>you</u> might behave, what <u>you</u> might be tempted to do.

• Listen as non-defensively as you can to any words of anger. If the feelings directed your way are justified, talk them through. Be genuine. If the feelings are really directed elsewhere but they happen to land on you, try not to take them personally. Be understanding.

• Take a break if you feel hurt or impatient or critical. Find ways to unwind.

Remind yourself what you already know: strong relationships can withstand difficult times. In fact, successfully navigating such times can make your relationships even stronger.

❁

6
Care for the other by caring for their environment.

People who are ill or incapacitated appreciate comfortable surroundings. They like to be in control of their environment as much as they're able. Most people prefer something home-like and personal. They also, more than not, like their setting to have signs of life and hope. As a caregiver, you can play a major role in helping to shape an environment that is pleasing, comforting, and fitting.

The atmosphere you help create and how you help create it will depend a great deal on the site. A healthcare facility will set certain bounds. Staff efficiency, infection control, and access to medical equipment are only a few of the factors determining the look and feel of those spaces. Some facilities can accommodate the preferences of patients and families more than others. Be sure to check first.

Most of the following suggestions apply to a person in a home setting, but some can be adapted to institutional use.

• A nearby telephone is usually desired. Would a portable phone or a speaker phone help?

• Contact with the outside world can be important. Any TV should be at a height they can easily see and the remote control needs to be at hand. A radio, newspapers, magazines, and books can provide additional information and entertainment.

• A bed table or lap desk will have untold uses.

• Writing materials for letters, notes, personal thoughts, and journaling can be placed within easy reach.

• For music lovers a tape deck or CD player can bring hours of pleasure.

• Pictures and mementos of loved ones, favorite places, and significant life events will lift spirits.

• Adequate sunlight really helps, as well as being able to rest directly in the sunlight a part of each day.

• Incandescent and natural lighting are kinder to the senses. Most fluorescent lighting is less so.

• Adequate moisture in the air and well-circulated air refreshes and cleanses.

• Affirming posters, pictures, and artwork can brighten the room and anyone within the room.

• Bringing nature's beauty inside is a healing act—things like plants, flowers, and other natural objects.

• A window that's easy to see can do wonders for one's healing. What about a bird or squirrel feeder just outside?

• Alternative "resting places" can offer choices of positions as well as scenery.

• A comfortable chair encourages relaxing visits with you or with others.

• The display of a symbol of one's faith may be appropriate.

• Fragrances and air fresheners can be renewing.

• If the other is an animal lover, consider making arrangements for a pet.

Remember there is an energy to a clean and orderly room. Re-arrange bed coverings and straighten personal effects from time to time. But place those effects to suit the other's tastes, not yours. And if the other wants things left exactly as they are, leaving them alone will be another way to show you care.

❀

7
Draw close to the other and the other's experience.

Some people feel uncomfortable around a person who is ill or disabled. It may show in their stilted conversation or by their obvious absence. It's not uncommon for some people to be in touch early in this experience and then have little or no contact afterwards, adding to the other's sense of loneliness and separation. That being the case, here are some ideas to keep in mind:

• People always appreciate reminders that others are keeping them close to heart. Cards, handwritten notes, small gifts, telephone calls, and short personal visits all convey that. Of all moments in your life together, this is the time to let the other know you care for them, and the ways you enjoy them.

• Most people like it when you come close physically. Touching the other as you greet them or leave them, or as you talk with them, can be confirming. Tender hugs can share both your caring and your energy.

• You may provide for the other's physical needs. If you're a full-time caregiver, that goes without saying. But even if you're a visiting friend or a "fill-in" caregiver, you might help with the other's hair or give them a manicure, a pedicure, a backrub, or a massage. When you give a massage, warm the lotion on your own hand first. Use slow, firm, consistent hand movements. When you've completed, don't withdraw your hands right away—stay in contact for several moments before gradually withdrawing your touch. The other will appreciate your gentleness and your sensitivity.

• If the other desires it, be close when their needs are greater—during pain or discomfort, when they're frightened, or when they cannot sleep.

• Deepen your closeness by encouraging the other not to feel guilty or upset about the inconveniences of your caregiving. Help them believe they would do as you have done, were the tables turned.

• You may be invited or you may volunteer to be a member of the other's medical team. In addition to medical caregivers, lay caregivers like yourself have a critical role to play. You can keep track of schedules, medications and other necessary recordkeeping. You can escort the other to doctor appointments and perhaps participate in those consultations. You can help remember both questions and concerns, both long words and little details, by taking notes or by carrying a tape recorder in those sessions. You can clarify hazy communications.

As a medical team member, you can serve a dual purpose that relates to the doctor or doctors. On the one hand, you can help the one in your care believe in their physician and in the information, advice, and expertise this person holds. Studies demonstrate that people with the greatest trust in their doctors tend to heal better and faster. On the other hand, you may serve a constructive purpose in de-mystifying the doctor, if that is needed. Your family member or friend may be hesitant to ask questions of the doctor, or to assert their right to have a certain minimal amount of the doctor's time. If there are concerns about the doctor's ability or advice, or about the chemistry between doctor and patient, you can help get a second or third medical opinion.

One final and critical factor about the other's medical team: one member of that team is more important than the rest–the one who is ill or incapacitated. That person has more at stake and possesses more knowledge of their internal condition than any of the rest of you. Treat that person accordingly.

❀

8
Establish boundaries.

You may have thoughts like these:

"Since the other person needs so much done, I'll do absolutely everything I can for as long as I can."

Or, "There is no one who understands this person as I do, and no one who can do what I can. So no one else will do those things but me."

Or, "Because the other person is so needy, I will do whatever they want, whenever they want, for as long as they want."

However admirable these thoughts appear, they can create problems for your caregiving. Here are two reminders:

• *You need to establish boundaries for your own good.*

Yes, it's true: you are needed. Yes, you can help, and yes, you may find meaning in doing that. But, no, you don't have to do it all. And, no, you don't have to do it to your own detriment.

Being always <u>with</u> another and doing constantly <u>for</u> another allows you no time to meet your own needs. And you have very important needs to be met. If you're not careful, you'll soon be on your way to exhaustion and burnout.

Some boundaries for you to set are physical. Some things are simply too strenuous for you to do. Some hours are too long for you to keep. Some chores you cannot continue to perform without relief.

Other boundaries for you to set are emotional. If you identify too completely with the other's pain or fear or other strong emotions, you will be in danger of making them your own. Your responsibility is to handle only one person's feelings: yours.

Remember also that setting limits to your caregiving will make room for more caregivers. Family members and friends may wish to share in these duties. It's one way they can cope with what has happened, and one way they can show their love.

• *You need to establish boundaries for the other person's good.*

One way you can respect the other is to give them their own space. They need their privacy just as before–perhaps to read or meditate or write. They may wish to look out the window and do nothing at all. If you do not provide for this solitary time, the one in your care may not have the strength or the heart to do so.

The other person needs the freedom to do things on their own as a matter of self-esteem, and perhaps for continued recovery. If you insist on doing too much, the other has too little opportunity to flex their muscles. And there are several kinds of muscles they may need to flex.

Good boundaries give this added benefit: you can be a more objective presence in their life. Your insight can be more accurate and your feedback can be more useful.

One final boundary you can provide is between the other and the outside world. Sometimes the one for whom you're caring is not ready to see certain people, or to be exposed to certain influences, or to be taxed by certain demands. You can help protect them, if that is what they wish.

All in all, establishing boundaries is one of the most thoughtful things you can do. It can even draw you closer together.

❀

9
Give good care to yourself
so you can be a good caregiver.

Concern for your personal care may seem selfish. But to place the other's needs automatically and continually before your own is an error—and a costly one.

However much you love the other person, you have only a certain amount of energy within your body. Once it's gone, it's gone. It does not magically replenish itself just because you wish it or the other person needs it.

There is only one way you can keep giving good care: you must have good care given to yourself on a regular basis. The one who is in the best position to provide that care is you. So your task is to make the nurturing you give yourself every bit as wholesome as the nurturing you give the other. When that happens, you can give better care for a longer period with more satisfaction. In a sense, therefore, caring for yourself is an act of unselfishness.

Among the various things you can do are these six:

• *Take care of your physical needs.* Eat well and drink wisely. Sleep all you need. Exercise regularly. Find ways to rest.

• *Protect yourself.* Reserve a period of time just for yourself at least once a day, and more often if you're able. Give yourself periods of time away, even longer periods. Restore yourself with brisk walks and with time spent in nature. Pursue whatever pastimes and hobbies you can.

• *Indulge yourself.* Give yourself small gifts that make you happy. Do things just for the fun of it. See if you can build a time of joy into every one of your days, something you can always look forward to.

• *Go easy on yourself.* Relax any self-imposed expectations that place unnecessary pressure on you or on others. Learn to be flexible. Speak accepting and affirming words to yourself.

• *Build a network of personal support.* Speak regularly with someone who cares and tell them what's going on with you. Talk about what it feels like to be in your position. Be with friends who cherish you and believe in you. Attend a support group if that sounds appealing. Take a class in caregiving if there is one in your community.

• *Allow others to help you.* When friends or neighbors say, "Let me know if there's anything I can do," let them know. Be appreciative of their offer and then be specific about what you need. Allow others to do some of your caregiving chores. If circumstances call for it, look into respite centers and other caregiver supports in your area. Turn to professionals when that's called for.

Ask for help when you need it. You may have to reverse some of your thinking about what it means to ask for this, and what it means when you receive it from others. You may be surprised what you discover. You may find that people are quite pleased to help–they just need your direction. You may find that more people are in a comparable situation than you realized. You may find that a true sense of community develops around you.

What you will find without question is this: the better care you give yourself, the better care you can give the other. The two go hand in hand.

❀

10
Relax into your role.

Caregiving, as you know, can be stress-producing. Being responsible for meeting another's needs can be a burden. When the other is quite ill or incapacitated, that burden can become terribly heavy. When most of the responsibility falls on one person's shoulders, the burden becomes heavier still.

You may be inclined to zero in on all the work that must be done. You may prepare to exert yourself and to labor, to knuckle down and to try hard. There is another way. You can relax.

• *You can relax into your body.* This is a time to make yourself comfortable. The more relaxed you feel, the more naturally you will function. If your caregiving is for a longer period of time, wear clothing that is easy to move around in. Pace yourself with how much you work and how fast you move. Learn some relaxation techniques if you don't know them already, and use them whenever you wish. Read an article or book on the subject–many are available. A healthcare professional can also advise you.

• *You can relax into your inner self.* Be as kind to your inner workings as you are to your outer being. Be accepting of whatever thoughts and feelings arise as a part of your caregiving. Allow them to surface and take notice of them. Let the warm and positive ones remain with you. Enjoy them. Share them if you wish. Should any uncomfortable reactions arise, take note of them as well. See what you can learn from them. Recognize them for what they are–feelings that are passing through, and thoughts that are meandering along. Then let them go.

Try some form of quiet meditation. Commune with your heart and your soul at least once a day and perhaps several times. Make this time as formal or as informal as you wish.

• *You can relax into your calling.* "Calling" may seem an unusual word for this work of yours, but it carries a truth. You have been called to this. Someone needed you and you are responding. Someone beckoned and you are answering.

No one called you to be Super Caregiver, however. You don't have to know everything and do everything and be everything. You'll learn and improve as time unfolds. Let that be enough. Be conscientious, but don't try to be perfect. Be something better—be human.

• *You can relax into your relationship with the other.* As you grow more calm within yourself and more comfortable in your role, you can become more at ease with the other. You learn to deepen your listening and to soften your touch. You learn to linger, without rushing to make everything right. For not everything can be made right. So you become that soothing presence that allows the other their pain, and in doing so, you make room for something more than the pain, for both of you.

"What am I to do," you may ask, "if I cannot relax into my role?" If, after giving yourself time and encouragement, it becomes clear that this role is not one you can comfortably assume, then you can do three things. You can arrange alternative ways to meet those caregiving needs, either with other volunteers or with professionals. You can continue to care for that person in ways that are less taxing for you. Finally, you can accept that the intimacy and immediacy of face-to-face caregiving is simply not your forte. You can understand that you are one of many like that, and that even though close caregiving is difficult for you, that does not mean you do not care. You can relax into a different style of caregiving.

❀

11
Accentuate the positive: catch joy, build belief, find hope.

This is a serious time in your life, and perhaps a sad time. You may be facing the unknown. Much may be at stake.

Whatever confronts you and whatever lies ahead for you, try to remember: these are not the only lasting realities in your life. Yes, it may seem so at the moment. You may find it hard to be optimistic. You may not feel like being upbeat. That's understandable.

Equally understandable is the fact that you cannot control what has happened, or what will happen. But this much you do have some control over: how you will respond. It is a control you alone can have. No one can give it to you, and no one can take it away from you.

• *It can help to look on the lighter side.* Sadness does not have to rule out every moment of joy. Seriousness does not bar all lightheartedness. It's possible still to smile and even joke.

You can do playful things for the other person. You can send funny cards, or read humorous books, or collect just the right jokes. You can bring audiotapes, videotapes, games, cartoons, and stories that add a sparkle to life. The two of you can watch a favorite TV comedy each time it's on. However these things benefit the other's spirits, they will benefit yours as well.

These need not be times of side-splitting laughter. Inside jokes, puns, and witty expressions can also be entertaining. Sometimes, in fact, you need not be funny at all. Just sharing quiet time together can be a very cheerful experience, for both of you.

• *It can help to enjoy whatever you find enjoyable.* There can be much to take pleasure in, if you're only open. Wherever you are and almost whatever you're doing, you can see things that comfort you or gladden you. You can be enchanted by what you hear, or fascinated by what you touch, or delighted by what you taste.

You can take satisfaction in the smaller things of life: children and animals, lighted candles and beautiful music, a favorite meal and a heartwarming memory. You may discover that the smaller things aren't so small after all.

• *It can help to emphasize the positive.* Even though you may not like all that's going on around you, you can choose what you will dwell upon and what you won't. You can decide whether you will mire yourself in all that's wrong, or encourage yourself with whatever can be right. You can concentrate on the awful or the awesome.

This does not mean hiding from the truth. It means assessing whatever truths are there and then selecting the truth upon which you will focus your energies.

• *It can help to believe.* This may be one of those times when the lessons of your faith come most poignantly alive. You may find that words of scripture, or hymns of assurance, or ancient stories of hope hold more meaning for you than ever before. You may experience deep satisfaction in knowing that others believe with you, whether they're members of your faith community, or participants in a prayer chain, or soulfriends of long-standing. You can also be inspired by the teachings of nature, by the examples of other people's lives, and even by the lessons being given you in this experience called "caregiving."

❀

12
Walk with the other in the search for meaning.

The other's illness is more than illness. The other's
surgery or injury or chronic disease or disability reaches
far beyond those experiences themselves. It pulls in the
person's self-image and their relationships with others,
especially loved ones. It pulls in their ideas about their
place in the world and their understanding of how the
world works. It pulls in their notions about work and
leisure, about what's important in life and what's "small
change."

Illness and incapacitation give one reason to pause and
to ask, "What am I to make of this? What meaning does
this hold for my life?"

Meaning is very personal. The meaning you make of
something may not be the same meaning someone else
would make of it. The significance you make of something today may not be the same you'll make of it
tomorrow. It may change and grow as you do.

Usually meaning takes time to discover. It takes
several opportunities to sort through and try on and test
out. It takes work. But finding meaning in life's events
is what can allow experiences that limit you to become
experiences that broaden you, however contradictory that
may seem.

The search for meaning is truly a search. You begin
without knowing exactly what you will find, or where or
when you will find it, or even if you will find it. That's
why the company of another can be helpful. That's why
there is value in the two of you walking together as you
hunt—you support the other person, and the other person
can support you. You each have meaning to find.

A good way to proceed is to ask a series of questions
and then see how the answers begin to form themselves.
Often they create their own pattern that becomes more

and more obvious in time. Questions you might talk about with the other person include these:

What have I learned about myself through this episode?

What have I learned about other people?

What do I now know about how I have related with other people in the past? About the way I relate to them today? About the way I want to relate in the future?

What has been taken away from me as a result of what has happened? What are the consequences of these losses?

What has been added to my life through this experience? What can I now do with those additions?

Are there ways I have grown as a result of what has happened to me? If so, what are those ways?

Is there any sense God has played a role in these events? If so, how? If so, what does that mean? If not, what does that mean?

What am I learning is most important in my life? What changes do I wish to make based on that importance?

The time the two of you spend together can be rich, as you discover new ideas, new learnings, and new meanings. In fact, the two of you can each discover a new "you."

❀

A Final Word ...

I once spoke about caregiving at a recognition banquet for medical caregivers. Afterward the husband of a nurse who was being honored requested a copy of my speech for himself. As I asked about his life, he explained he had a severely handicapped teenage son who could not walk and could barely talk. This father did much of the day-to-day care, since the boy was too big for the mother to lift. He even took his son to work with him every day and watched over him in the back of his jewelry shop.

"Until I heard your talk this evening," he said, "I had never thought of myself as a caregiver."

I was stunned at his admission. I have since heard similar words many times. Too often people who are not professional caregivers do not see themselves as real caregivers. Perhaps you are like that. Perhaps you doubt the validity or the importance of what you do.

If you're like most family and volunteer caregivers I know, you regularly perform work that goes unnoticed and unappreciated. You put aside your own desires for the good of someone else. You willingly do chores you don't like. You expertly wear many hats at the same time. And you do all this with a humility and a grace that belies how difficult your role truly is.

I, and many others, salute you.

❁

An Affirmation of Those Who Care for Others

I believe in the power and the beauty of self-forgetful love,
and further I believe it shows itself right in our midst.
It is offered by family members and by friends,
by volunteers and by professionals alike,
as they tenderly care for those
who suffer illness, injury, or incapacitation.
I believe this unassuming selflessness comes to life
each time someone looks after another,
despite feeling winded or weary;
each time someone manages countless caregiving details,
all in addition to their other daily obligations;
each time someone performs duties of care freely out of love
that others would not perform for a much higher price.
I believe these openhearted spirits are a model for all of us.
For they show us the potential of what life can be:
In quietly persevering with another,
life can be vitalized and expanded.
In patiently witnessing what another is experiencing,
life can be deepened and ennobled.
And in lovingly accepting how the other is coping,
life can be strengthened and enriched.
I believe that in their learning, we are taught.
We are taught that remaining faithfully with another who suffers
is more than an act of compassion—it is a ritual of healing.
We are taught that reaching out to another who feels isolated and alone
is more than a bridge of comfort—it is a sacrament of communion.
We are taught that relating to the other as a person of infinite value
is more than an article of faith—it is the lived experience of sacredness.
We know that because others have shared themselves openly,
and life is not the same: not for them, not for us,
and especially not for those who are bathed in this generous care.

—James E. Miller

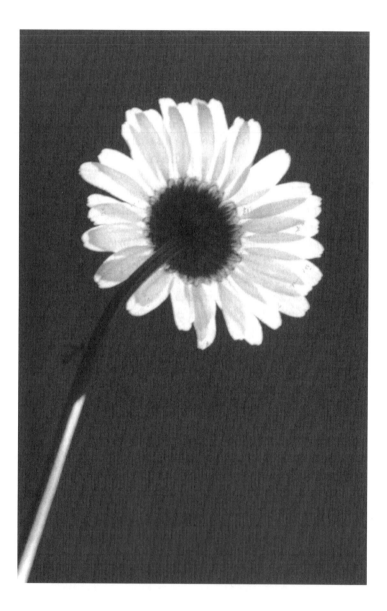

Remember that as you help another toward healing and wholeness,
you are helping yourself toward that same goal.